Reflections

New and Selected Poems

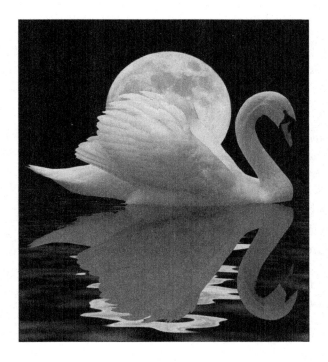

Ute Carson

Plain View Press, LLC
www.plainviewpress.net

1101 W 34th Street STE 404
Austin, TX 78705

ISBN: 978-1-63210-032-0
Library of Congress Control Number: 2018933167

Cover art
Reflected Swan © David Benton | Dreamstime.com
File ID: 4254722 License: Royalty Free
David Benton: ttps://www.dreamstime.com/spurious2_info

The Moon © Thomas Lammeyer | Dreamstime.com
File ID: 2825480 License: Royalty Free
Thomas Lammeyer: https://www.dreamstime.com/lammeyer_info

Cover design by Pam Knight
Author photo by Jeffery Powers

We Find Healing In Existing Reality

Plain View Press is a 40-year-old issue-based literary publishing house. Our books result from artistic collaboration between writers, artists, and editors. Over the years we have become a far-flung community of humane and highly creative activists whose energies bring humanitarian enlightenment and hope to individuals and communities grappling with the major issues of our time—peace, justice, the environment, education and gender.

for my family

Acknowledgements

Gratitude to the following publications for previously publishing these poems:

"Old Age, Another Country" (*Scissors and Spackle*, Vol. 3, November 2011)

"The Waters Within" (*Scissors and Spackle*, Vol. 4, December 2011)

"Nostalgic Summer Days" (*Everyday Poems*, October 2011)

"A Tangled Nest of Moments" Second Place in the Eleventh International Poetry Competition, (*Firstwriter Magazine*, UK, 2011)

"The Mysteries of Others" (*GringolandiaSantiago*, January 2012)

"Give me a Grandparent" (*GringoLandiaSantiago*, May 2012)

"Whiskers in the Night" (*CatTales V*, May 2012)

" Milk and Tears" and "Let There Be Light" (*Rusty Nail Magazine*, June 2012)

"Homecoming" (*Riverlit Magazine*, Vol. 7, August 2012)

"In a Bubble of Bliss" (*The Green Silk Journal*, Spring Issue 2012)

"Bodies in Mourning" (*Misfits Miscellany Magazine*, September 2012)

"Toward Evening" and "Generational Window-Watching" (*Attitude and Culture Journal of Crimean Tatars*, Rumania 2012)

"Folding Washing", "Morning Ritual" and "Nothing in Nature Is Ever Lost" (*Gravel Magazine*, August 2013)

"Remains of a Life", "Elegy for a Dying Friend", "The Family Album", "Grief", "The Space Between", "Combustible", "You Could Be Wrong" and "Living Deferred" (*Folding Washing*, The Willet Press, 2013)

"Binding the Years" (*The Green Silk Journal*, Spring Issue 2013)

"Messengers" (*Lone Star Magazine*, Issue 74, January 2013)

"Today's Slippers Become Tomorrow's Army Boots" (*Morgan Bailey's Writing Blog*, May 2013)

"Eternity" and "Once More for Real" (*My Gift to Life*, Rumania, 2014)

"Time Past, Time Present" (*Ariadne's Thread Literary Magazine*, Issue 14, Winter 2014/15)

"Unique Beauty of an Old Face" (*Poppy Road Review*, May 2015)

"Extra Padding" and "Sunrise/Sunset" (*The Greenwich Village Literary Review*, Vol. II, No. 1, Spring 2015)

"Time Stands Still" (*Mother's Milk Books Writing Prize*, Anthology 2015)

"Before the Traces are Lost" and "In My End Is My Beginning" (*Nazar Look Magazine*, Issue 45, Winter 2015)

"Waiting" (*TRACKS*, Inwood Indiana Press, 2016)

"Tree Forks" (*Evening Street Press*, Vol. 14, Spring 2016)

"Now" (*Mother's Milk Books Writing Prize*, Fall 2016)

"Chambers of My Heart", "Mystery", "I Love You Even More" and "Lemonade" (*The Aras and Jasmine Journal*, Winter 2016)

"When Did I Get Old? (*Stark, The Poetry Journal, Wisehouse International Poetry Award*, No. 1, 2016)

"Reaching for the Morning Star", "Time, the Mother of Transformation", "The Scarf" and "Riding the Coattails of the Morning Sun" (*Longshot Island Magazine*, February 2017)

"Seven Decades On", "Bow and Arrow" and "More than Memorabilia" (*Once Written Magazine*, UK, May 2017)

"Old Heart" (*Greensilk Journal*, May 2017)

Contents

Tree Forks

Let There Be Light

for Dylan

It's the attentive hour
when the world dances
with glorious fires of sunsets
before darkness extinguishes
the last wondrous glow
on the quivering horizon.

Wise owl, bird of the night,
watchful eyes sharply focused,
keen ears perked,
will soon tune in
to whispers of loneliness,
shrieks of fear,
and gasps of grief.

Rapt in terrified awe
by the moon's beguiling glare,
we wait for a different dance
to move us though the hours of gloom
toward a flickering sky,
igniting into a daylight candle.

Nostalgic Summer Days

A cluster of dark trees
blurring into a green knoll,
emerald sheen on velveteen moss,
sprays of daisies across the grass,
bees greedily drinking from succulent centers,
quick-stepping deer flitting by,
fallen feathers of magpies.
Naked feet dangle in a silvery brook
that licks our soles with its babbling tongue,
and we children lapse into repose.

Spider-leafed shadows
of late afternoon
as light is drained from the sky
inhabit me.
Lush blueberries brim
over the rim of my basket.
Our laughter leaves me breathless.
I close my eyes.
My life is strongly scented
with the happiness of childhood.

Mother of Many Children

There is no fairest of them all!
Cradling a new baby in my arms
I was flooded with a bounteous thankfulness.
Over the years more offspring arrived,
the next generation.

Now each time I hold a little one
an inexhaustible spring
of maternal love bubbles up again
and I baptize them all
with my eternal gratitude.

In a Bubble of Bliss

for Kaius

In the cradle of my arms
I safeguard my baby's sleep,
and my emotions envelop my heart
in a snug embrace.
For a while, before the baby wakes,
I live in a bubble of bliss.

Each awakening is a leaving.
Children carry the ball of life forward,
run with it, make goals, miss targets,
fumble it, kick it in disappointment,
and toss it in and out of relationships.
They move on
and their future rolls out of my sight.

Until one day, unexpectedly,
a child or grandchild turns around
and throws the ball backwards.
"Catch, Mama."
"Catch, Omi."
For a moment I live again
in a bubble of bliss.

Ute Carson

Time Stands Still

for Lucas and Kaius

New life flows through my tiny grandson,
its course unknown to me.
What I do know is the feeling
of his warm body nestled against mine
like a small animal,
heart to heart, rapid beats to my sluggish rhythms.

And I know bliss
lying with his brother
in grass as high as our mounts' manes
gently combed by an autumn breeze,
frogs croaking in the shimmering algae on the pond,
and him asking, "Can we stay here all day? And swim?"

Trust

Baby arms slung around my neck,
fuzzy head slumped against my shoulder,
or a toddler's hand pressed securely into mine.
For a parent, a loving responsibility,
for a child a trust fund
to draw on for the rest of its life.

Lemonade for Sale

My sister is six, I am eight,
and today we will earn our first money
from fresh-squeezed juice sweetened with honey.
Dad has laid a board across cement blocks.
Mother gave us plastic cups and a faded blue ceramic pitcher.
Our sign announces in big yellow letters,
"LEMONADE 10 CENTS A GLASS."
Our piggybanks—a sleek wooden whale
and a round pink porcelain chicken—
are perched on the little stand
and we are open for business.
As cars approach, slow down, then speed up again
we wave and shout,
"Lemonade for sale here, lemonade."

Tree Forks

On an ultrasound my uterus resembles the Tree of Life.
In its blood-paneled enclosure
my children were all mine.
Outside the womb they put down roots in different soils,
leafing out on branches of their own.
My sap still seeps through their arteries and veins
but I can no longer nourish their growth
or give them shelter.

How far has the fruit fallen?
Goethe wrote: "We cannot shape our children in our image.
We must love them as God gave them to us,
bring them up as best as we can, and then let them be."
With the passage of time fresh starts blossom,
trembling with shades of rainbow colors,
and spreading their unique fragrances
while the old tree shakes its dusky leaves with pride.

Ute Carson

The Scarf

My daughter has knitted me a lilac mohair scarf
with swishing tassels along its ends.
"It was a struggle," she says, "to make love more than momentary."
She began with a simple left-to-right pattern,
then added a spidery loop here and there.
She had to unravel and start again more than once.

Now the shawl reaches down to my waist
revealing complex needle maneuvers,
ridges alternating with smooth stretches.
When I envelop myself in this precious gift,
I feel my daughter's presence
woven into every stitch.

This Is the Life

Aging can be a time of freedom
to cherish the pitter-patter of grandchildren,
to see your own face, mirrored and wrinkled,
confront you with an obstinate smile,
to watch the green ear of a plant
eagerly forging up through crusted soil.
Aging also requires courage
not to give up on an unwilling mind,
not to mourn the failings of your body.
But when my lover
takes my hand in his,
I know this is the life.
I would want no other.

The Family Album

for Nicholas

It feels as though dust and cobwebs
are swirling around me
as I paste faded black and white photographs
into albums.
I label them all with names and dates,
rolling back the years to bygone generations.
There are pictures of many family events,
moments of lives captured with a simple click.
I know my relatives from their stories
and the traits they left behind,
grandpa's temper, my uncle's sullen disposition.
Their gestures reveal something of their character,
sitting ramrod straight, hands clasped over knees,
a mouth raised slightly at the edges.
Inherited looks glimpsed in my mother's eyes,
green-blue, the color of rainwater
now sparkle in my daughter's eyes, and
my own skin is furrowed like my grandmother's.
But the intimacies of life are missing.
My ancestors were once flesh-and-blood,
now silence surrounds them monk-like.
I wish I could query my parents
about their dreams and defeats.
When I was young I showed little interest
and now they are no longer here to be asked.
Wisdom and insight are so often delayed.
I enter a mysterious territory of inferences,
land of the imagination,
as I try to spool back the years.
A veil stretches over the lives of my family
and when I lift the hem
I see only snapshots, frozen in time.

Give Me a Grandparent

On her wedding day my daughter turned to me
and said, "Thank you for giving me a grandmother."

Through tranquility and turmoil
grandparents bridge the decades
as the oil in their lamps burns low,
their lives no longer in constant motion,
and time is measured by the fleeting seasons.
Grandparents have ears like conch shells
echoing the wishes and woes of the young.
With hearts galvanized by patience and necessity,
they try to protect the next generation
from their own youthful follies.

Grandchildren fritter away time
as if they had a thousand years.
But the young are free to lay claim to the old.
Together they can peer at the man in the moon,
weave dreams on a magic carpet,
buy the bra that can't yet be filled,
welcome the strangely attired boyfriend,
and use those ready-made laps as safe perches
when thunder claps and lightning strikes.

Grandparents sing songs
they have stored up inside them
so that their beloved grandchildren can dance.

Generations

for Zachary

On our wide bed my grandson slumbers deep in dreams,
his right leg tossed over my left hip,
his arms linked around my neck.
I inhale his sweet toddler breath
and wish that, holding him tight,
the world could be condensed
into this wondrous sensation.
Love between grandparents and grandchildren
is easy, taken for granted,
the one receiving unconditional acceptance,
the other the satisfaction of being needed.

Generational Window-Watching

Outside his window
the snowflakes descend light as dust,
slowly falling through endless distance.
The old man rocks rhythmically,
curled up in a comforter like a hibernating animal.
His gaze glides over the glacier-blue scenery below.
Wasn't it just yesterday that he shoveled snow
into waist-high drifts along the driveway?
He muses as a sparrow dashes to the wooden feeder
swinging from an adjacent tree branch.
The old man reposes in silence
knowing that in another season
he can observe the rebirth of a flowering earth.

Years ago on a chilly morning
he dashed to the bedroom window in his pajamas
and pressing his nose against the frosted glass
breathed a peek-hole into a magical world,
silvery under the early light.
It had snowed and the garden, deep in winter sleep,
was as unblemished as his young life.
A rabbit scurried from under a frost-sugared bush
and left paw prints on the white ground.
In his excitement the boy wanted nothing more
than to run after the wild creature.
In a voice a trifle too high he called to his mother,
"Let's go down. I want to touch."

Now the coltishness of his youth long gone,
movements have slowed,
this wordless watching
replaces his impatient exuberance with aged admiration
as a cardinal flits by,
the evening sun red on its underwings.

Ute Carson

The Space Between

Watching My Mother

My mother and I share a room tonight.
I look at her, curled onto her side,
her furrowed brow relaxed.

Already I'm having second thoughts
about having asked if I could wear earplugs
to muffle her snoring.
This morning at breakfast
I pointed out a morsel of food
clinging to a corner of her mouth,
wishing she had noticed it herself.
And I grew so irritated when she told
the pious ladies at today's luncheon,
who thanked their heavenly father for his blessings,
that after Auschwitz one can no longer
count on a caring God.

Now that my mother is deep in slumber,
I feel tender remorse tightening my chest.

Now

Breathless he runs toward his teammates
who call out, "C'mon, let's play!"
He dashes past his grandmother
who sits expectantly on a bench
and reaches out from habit
to touch his sleeve,
"Not now," he frowns.

He sees the disappointment on that beloved face.
For a split second, stories, songs and games
embedded in his memories of childhood
make him feel that he should go back,
say something to her,
though he is not sure what.
Instead he rushes on to where he wants to be, now.

Ute Carson

The Space Between

After school you jumped into the car,
gushing like an open water hose
with news of the day,
"We released the butterflies...." "Jackie hit me...."

Today it's phone calls and text messages,
a stopover between planes,
long distance communications,
"Hope you're doing alright...all's well here...."

First you were loved,
so you learned to love,
you were cared for
and you've become a caring person.

What do I miss?
Once there was little space between us,
narrow as a needle's eye,
through which whispers could be threaded.

Bow and Arrow

Letting my children go
was like throwing open a pigeon coop.
They flew in all directions
and I fluttered right behind them
cooing, cajoling, corralling, counseling
and watching with pride as they built their own nests.

Now that the grandchildren are fledglings
a different image flashes before me.
I am holding a bow,
the string is taut
and though my hand is steady and my eyes are focused,
my stomach is twisted into anxious knots.

As I let the arrow fly, my gaze follows its course
until it vanishes from sight.
I stay rooted to the ground,
no longer able to fly along.
My heart contracts. I hope
I have infused the slender missile with all my love.

Ute Carson

Waiting

for Alexander

I wait for many things:
For snow to melt,
for God to answer a question
for my lover to declare his intentions,
for my body to heal.
But Sunday mornings
I listen for the phone to ring
so that a grandchild's voice,
travelling over great distances,
can bring me joy that lasts
long after the conversation ends.

Today's Slippers Become Tomorrow's Army Boots

Warm bodies, heated anticipation
fuse our solidarity.
Snug in knitted booties
we stretch out on our magic carpet,
the children young, content as kittens.
I orchestrate flights of fancy
and promise the little ones
that the swords and crowns missing by morning
will reappear come dreamtime.

Years later,
a grandson walks down his childhood path,
boots shining with confidence,
but the back of his grey coat
bars me from seeing through to his heart.
My hands fling forward wanting to hold on
but I pull back,
my fears cling to my upturned palms.

We lose our children to the world
which shapes them beyond our wishes and control.
Proudly we teach them
to be self-sufficient
but we never learn not to worry.

Ute Carson

You Can't Earn It

Love is like the lucky penny you happen upon,
the clearing you spy
beyond a forest thicket.
If you only reach into your own pocket
no love token will be found.
No thank-yous may ever arrive
for the love gifts you send.
But if you become like "Sterntaler,"*
giving freely and expecting nothing,
a shower of stars may sprinkle down upon you.

*A poor homeless girl with a big heart gives her only loaf of bread to a
hungry man and the clothes she wears to needy children. With nothing
left to give, stars fall at her feet, becoming talers. And she finds herself
clothed in fine linen.
    Grimms' Fairy Tales

Chambers of My Heart

My heart has many chambers.
Lodgers come and go, often
leaving something of themselves behind.
Others just move on.
Only one is allowed
to roam from room to room.
My heart harbors a secret hope
that he will like my place so much
he will claim it and move in.

Octopus

Sometimes I wish I was an octopus
with several arms and legs.
Instead I have only two legs,
but that is all I need to run to you,
and two arms only,
quite enough
to hold you close.

Messengers

Naked feet carry me to your bed,
quicksilver words whisper in your ear,
my soft voice quickening your dreams,
and my drowsy eyes spirit your troubles away.
But it is my hands that offer love.
When I squeeze your hand
my hand holds the memory
of yours all through the day,
and at night I reach out
to touch it again.

Morning Ritual

I used to bolt from bed
as if my bag of duties
had to be delivered
before the sun burned through the haze.

Now I move over to you
on the pillow next to mine.
Curled around each other,
our warmth mingles.

When the cock crows
and day dawns
we roll out together
hip-to-hip.

Binding the Years

Homecoming

He is bathed in the blue luster of the porch light,
hair tousled, cheeks cross-hatched with lines,
the knot in his throat tight,
balancing a glass of wine in each hand,
and music from inside the house
beguiling the late hour.

Every Thursday evening
she slides from their worn old truck,
yoga bag slung over her left shoulder,
her right hand gripping the door handle.
Raindrops tap her face,
foretaste of his welcoming kiss.

"I'm home," her voice muffled in the mist.
But he hears.
Always the vaguely anxious anticipation,
then relief.
He is waiting, she is back.
When the heart grows older
there is much to lose.

I Love You Even More

New relationships sparkle and glitter,
they can be exciting adventures
treading virgin ground
on the lookout
for chance encounters.

Old relationships have a history,
they are seasoned by experience.
Couples bound by years
may amble along a smoother path,
savoring a layered, deeper love.

Ute Carson

River of Life

I wade at the bend in the River
where it narrows before widening.
A cool breeze swirls around my ankles.
I am at midpoint between the trickle from a spring
and the final emptying into the ocean.
I listen to the River, a talker,
and try to block the universal wailing,
the human misery coloring the water blood-red.

Then out of a foamy pool
a water lily rises,
blowing bubble kisses through the spray.
My heart leaps to grasp the glistening blossom.
But in no time the rushing current greedily
sucks the flower under
and the waves crush it against the shore,
wickedly flashing their crests like deadly knives.

Binding the Years

I catch a whiff of childhood,
the little girl of my memory,
hand-in-hand with her mother,
a cherub with a dazzling smile.

The woman of my middle years I know best,
confidence encircling her like perfume,
and stumbling head over heels
into good fortune and follies.

I feel tender toward my old self,
the woman with the weather-worn face,
faltering steps, swaying from side to side,
and lifelong stored-up insights.

I am reminded of a bunch of dandelions,
turning from golden blossoms
into fluffy silver seeds
about to be winged away by a boisterous wind
in directions unknown.

Ute Carson

Reaching for the Morning Star

for Lucas

Two year-old Lucas doesn't know
that without my morning Advil
gravity would pull my aging body down
so that my arms could not spread wide in greeting
when his radiant person bounds through the door.

Snuggled on his grandpa's lap
Lucas doesn't know
that his beloved reader's old heart
sometimes skips and jumps more wildly
than the monkeys in the storybook.

When he tosses his head back and says "catch me"
Lucas can't know
that my feet feel stuck as though in sand.
Hopping like a rabbit up the stairs, he giggles
as I creep up behind him at a snail's pace.

Our little grandson is carefree and safe with us,
enveloped in our seasoned love,
and he in turn inspires us every day,
even after a sleepless night,
to get up and reach for the morning star.

Riding the Coattails of the Morning Sun

Like a knob-kneed colt
with wild mane flying
I galloped carefree through my youth.
Muddy potholes and thorny hedges
were no obstacles but welcome challenges.
Sparks flew from my radiant body
as I rode on the coattails of the morning sun.

Now I sit by candlelight,
a crocheted comforter around my shoulders,
recalling old wrongs and shortcomings
as well as the delicate beauties of my life
--and tell stories.

Ute Carson

Old Age, Another Country

I want to get off that fast train
that makes no leisurely stops
at quaint country stations
to let me cross the tracks
and ride back.

I have packed the wrong books,
my tailored suit pinches my waist,
my ankles are swollen,
and my hair is a frizzle
from a nocturnal rumble through memories.

I thought myself prepared.
Loved ones assured me that
this journey would be manageable.
Now I sulk with a headache
and the cold station sandwich sits in my stomach
like a sack of wet grain.

I try to adjust,
use my jacket as a pillow,
drink in the passing landscape
with longing eyes,
suppressing the urge to jump out
and run light-footed across the blooming meadows
with the sun tickling my nose.

I feel confined
but hope that when I reach my destination
I will find something pleasant and familiar
in a country I have no desire to visit.

When Did I Get Old?

Age crept up on me like a mist over clear water.
In a snapshot taken from a distance
blurred by years,
the outlines are still visible.
My posture exudes the confidence
my mother praised in her "little princess."
Joyful pride radiates from my body,
knowing how hard it worked
as a lover and a mother.

I like my wrinkles best.
A lot of experience is etched into those lines.

Zooming in for a close-up,
I can't recall when I added a double chin,
or plush cushions around my once slender waist.
And how could my swollen feet glide across a dance floor?
But then I see a photograph of
my husband's broad hand with sun-flaked skin
spread protectively over my small crooked hand
covered with ladybug spots,
and I think, "It is what it is, and it's not so bad."

Ute Carson

Seven Decades On

When I'm eighty I don't want people to say,
"You're looking younger every day."
Or "You don't look your age at all!"
I want them to say that I am beautiful
like a winter rose holding its petals snug,
brilliant as I was in the greenness of spring,
the full-blooming summer,
and the gold-wilting fall.

Extra Padding

Shrinkage of mind and decline of body
suggest that we shrivel and wilt.
Instead, as we grow older,
we become plump
like overripe fruit.
Is it the cold north wind
rustling our memories,
or daily tasks rattling our weary bones
that make extra padding
a necessary protection for the old?

Ute Carson

Unique Beauty of an Old Face

Praises are sung of the rosebud faces of youth
but little is said about a face with lifelines.
The bold reds of former years
have given way to silvery hair
that surrounds her face like in a cloud of wisdom.
Her lips have narrowed and lost their fullness,
but they speak truthfully,
having little to hide.
Sorrow and joy are furrowed into her cheeks,
crisscrossing them like a plowed field.
And her eyes? What have they not seen?
These sea-colored globes quiver
with her soul's struggles and triumphs.
Her face no longer gleams with innocence and wonder
but with a refined radiance
born of life's hard-won experiences.

Folding Washing

Old Heart

Lub dup. lub dup. lub dup,
muscles flex, soundwaves murmur
day by day, year after year.
You never let me down.
Loves flowed freely in and out of
your crimson chambers as welcome guests.
When they departed there were hugs
and sometimes tears
but you never missed a beat.
You were ageless then.

There are fewer guests now.
Your walls have thinned,
your rhythms slowed, your beats labored.
Still one lifelong love
you cling to with every tenuous sinew,
anxious that you might shut down
should that guest ever leave.

Be brave, old heart.
Let even your most precious love
come and go
as if you were still young
with nothing to fear,
as if the heart could never stop.

Folding Washing

"...*Grow Old With Me*
The Best Is Still To Be..."

It's hard to believe the promise
when aging's afflictions begin to weigh on us,
the failing body, the forgetful mind.
But if we're lucky
we'll have someone to fold washing with,
long sheets needing two pairs of hands,
tugging, straightening,
stretch right, pull to the left.
The heart will not be deterred,
forever yearning for a companion
to share the ordinary
with lightness as dusk descends.

Ute Carson

Old Couples

Old couples hold hands.
They don't stop on the main plaza to kiss
or lose themselves in embraces on park benches.
Like elephants they tread in each other's footsteps,
aware of frailty but steady and confident.
Young couples resemble cats,
tails intertwined, purring.
But once they spot a scurrying mouse,
they jump in fresh hot pursuit.

Alone But Not Lonely

In my feverish delirium
I long for the cool hand of my lover,
a balm on my forehead.
We share life's journey
but the frayed nerves and fearful dreams
are now mine alone.

My parents rejoiced together at my birth,
but I had to squirm from darkness into light
to suck in that first breath myself.

I hope that when I lie dying,
arms will hold me
and lips whisper farewell kisses.
Still, only I can sever
the umbilical cord to the world.

To prepare for the day
when the place next to me
is vacant, I treasure
the fleeting security of togetherness.

Ute Carson

Time Past, Time Present

There is a battered trunk in the attic
containing my world of yesteryear.
I have lived fully but unreflectively
and the gifts I was given
found their way into the chest,
taken for granted as life hastened on.

Now as I grow old
I lift them out one by one
and gingerly hold them up
to the soft silver light of sunset
which illuminates them with a clarity
I had not seen before
in the blinding sunrays of dawn.

Time, Mother of Transformation

I cradle the old man in his dying,
his rough stubble brushes my arm.
He drools like my teething eight-month old.
Did he once snuggle against his mother's breast?
Before he lost lucidity he told me
he had been a shepherd roaming the Highlands
with his dog Benno.
"One nod of my head and off he went
to bring in the flock."
Now the old man only mumbles,
"I had a little lamb, its fleece as white as snow."

Ute Carson

The Power of Words

The Word became flesh,
living flesh, commanding, knowing.
Like wind travelling along telephone wires
words rush over sound waves of joy, sorrow and anger.
Words define us.
Beware of words!
Once spoken, regret cannot retrieve them.
Believe in words!
"I am leaving" might mean just that,
               but
"I love you" may have the power
to move the heart.

More Than Memorabilia

Special objects hold time.
People live on in them.

The silver-plated brush
with yellowed bristles
stroked my grandmother's long black hair.
A lipstick imprint on the rim
of my mother's dainty porcelain cup
recalls years of afternoon teas.
The soft threads in my lover's sweater
carry his familiar scent.
Numerous love-worn toys and books
tell of children and grandchildren.

Such objects gleam with meaning,
bring consolation,
allow us to live with death,
and ground us
in the here and now.

Ute Carson

Whiskers in the Night

We buried our beloved old cat
next to our bedroom window
under the sway of roses,
close to the roaming ivy
which will soon cover his resting place.

Moons later the night pulses with dim starlight
and the wind utters surly sighs of annoyance
while our house is solemn with sleep.
I perk up my ears as the windowpane rattles
and a wobbly shadow floats out of the dark earth
with a rustling sound similar to a finger
running along the bristles of a comb.
Our cat purred like that.
When I glance up at our bedroom ceiling
painted yellow by crooked moonbeams,
fluid lines, curled like whiskers, spin
and their reflections spiral downward
to a spot on the bed once reserved for our agile cat.
I reach for the black and white wisps,
now dancing imprints on the sheet,
swirling into a fur-ball.
But my touch comes away empty
and I wake with a vague longing.

As darkness melts and pale sunrays crawl
into the spaces of the curtain,
daylight rearranges my thoughts
and an echo from the night reverberates.
I rush to the window.
In the dew-moistened bushes
raindrops glisten on whiskers.
A beckoning meow,
a message from our old companion?

Grief

Loss,
the most violent storm she will ever encounter,
winging away her loved one beyond arms' reach.
She stumbles, doubles over,
tears like acid scalding her face.
She sinks to the ground without volition,
her fingers clawing the blood-soaked earth.
Nothing can make it better,
and nothing holds any worth.
Then with time a hedge grows
out of rubble and sticks,
and sprigs leaf out into myriad arms
which take the form of a soft white kitten,
letters from friends, consoling hugs.
And as the arms weave a web of compassion,
they rock her grief-stricken soul
and tenderly embrace her bruised body
until the storm loses its hold.
Then the arms relax,
releasing the convalescent once more
back onto life's familiar shore.

Ute Carson

Elegy for a Dying Friend

Swans sing a song before dying.
Now in my friend's avian garden
many birds have assembled,
making music to ease her departure.

A couple of classy cardinals chirp in rhyme,
a hummingbird light as a butterfly
twitters in exaltation like a lark.
Two tiny Carolina wrens with big voices
strike up a new melody
as a crow caws and scolds.
Then three blue jays,
in flight looking for bugs,
add their pearly sounds.
Nearby a peep of chickens clucks,
a rooster croaks huskily,
and a muster of pheasants pleasantly chortles
as peacocks shriek, loud and less charming.
The mystical distelfink,
bird of love and longevity, mates in the air,
emitting cries of joy.

My friend finds completeness
listening to the cacophony of birdsong,
knowing that soon she too will take flight.
Death can only touch what life has touched.
What will she sing?

Milk and Tears

Sprouting from sturdy shoulder blades
my arms branch out into huge angel-wings.
One wing is bridal-veil white,
its feathers dotted with tiny pearls
quietly pouring sweet breast milk
into the expectant mouths of babes.
The other wing is black crepe
loudly fluttering in the howling wind,
bone shafts filled with tears,
spilling over from suffering and loss.
Now both wings flap vehemently
like kites about to soar,
and I feel like a great blue heron on spindly legs
gracefully unfurling heavy plumage
then lifting off,
trying my best
to keep my angel-wings in balance.

Ute Carson

Bodies in Mourning

In the waiting room of the dying
bodies clad in sadness
make last statements
as time runs out
like sand in an hourglass.
They sit on chairs facing each other,
sewing shrouds,
thread whispering through cloth,
weaving light and dark hues into the fabric
for lives lived or unclaimed.

Anemic blood,
broken capillaries on skin,
dry vaginas,
slack penises,
drum-bellied growling guts,
fading hearts,
try to muffle the voice of death.
All the while,
earthbound flesh longs for weightlessness.

Other bodies wean themselves
slowly from life,
revisit bygone places,
reconnect with long-lost loves,
relive past pleasures.
Tremors of yearning
still pulse through veins worn thin,
and unquenched desire burns in old eyes,
until a gentle breeze
snuffs out the last labored breath
and sends parting puffs of gratefulness
into the smoky air.

Once More for Real

Nothing in Nature Is Ever Lost

She slips into dying like the setting sun.
Only slowly does she notice the change
as those around her fall silent.
An old woman's loneliness.
She long ago abandoned the belief
that God's eye is on her as on a sparrow,
but she still puts the best of herself
onto the enduring pages of her diary,
confessing her sleeping potion
of lukewarm water with shots of whisky
and her dreams of dark shadows flitting by.
But when the stars dim
and a faint pink line brightens the horizon,
and her dog nudges her to be let out,
she makes her way
to the crumbling backdoor steps,
folding her aging flesh beneath her
and sips soothing tea through her thin lips.
Her teaming garden,
bougainvillea cascading water-like over the fence
is not a bad place to contemplate dying,
birds stirring in the bushes,
dragonflies skimming the grass
sweet with dew as though rinsed by tears.
She inhales wild mint-scented air.
When she tilts her head back she can see the sky,
and only slowly pulls in her wings,
knowing that the earth is gentle
to all living things that fall into her embrace
to be harbored and to await germination
for the annual rebirth.

Remains of a Life

He is buried and the entire sale is over.
Paintings have been shipped to a gallery,
books donated to the local library,
antique furniture sent to a dealer for appraisal.
The grandchildren salvaged some treasures,
the Wedgewood china, a silver tea set,
a Gone-with-the-Wind lamp,
and some colorful Venetian glassware.
Then for three days strangers' feverish hands
pawed through boxes, spread piles across the lawn
like an angry wind scattering whatever was loose.
Now there are only
a few items for the Salvation Army,
a rickety armchair, a battered wooden trunk,
picnic chairs stacked on a picnic table,
a mouse-gray teddy bear,
a wallet stuffed with pictures
and clothes strewn about like so much debris.
Sadness washes over me.
All these objects once had a life of their own,
a power, a language.
They had been needed, collected, cherished.
I dab my eyes on my sleeve,
overcome by the unbridgeable separateness
between the living and the dead,
and fervently hope that
the deceased took memories of beautiful objects
and meaningful moments with him
and stored them forever in his soul.

Ute Carson

Eternity

Amidst life's clamor
I cannot imagine the silence
that will one day surround me.
I will not hear the footfalls above me,
nor feel the rain weeping on my grave.
I will not be able to thank a grandson
for bringing me flowers
or wipe away a granddaughter's tears
as she kisses the stone face
on which my name is engraved.

But within earshot of my lover
I fervently hope
that my whispers will meet his
through the roots and tendrils
of porous earth
and we will gurgle and murmur
like two underground streams
which know nothing of endings.

Once More for Real

Now that I have children
and grandchildren of my own,
the beloved faces of my childhood
emerge from the past
as through a clearing in the mist
and explode into light.
The fragrance of my mother's sweet perfume
as her lullabies fill my dreams.
My father's stories resurfacing
from the deep recesses of my mind.
Even my childhood dog's cold nose
rubbing against my cheek
reawakens vivid joys.
If memory is alive
the dead are alive.
If only I could hug them
once more for real.

Ute Carson

Reflections on a Journey

Where there is an ending
there was a beginning
when anticipation quarreled with apprehension.
Now memories sift through moments in the journey.
Though we walked along roughly pebbled roads
we found many gold nuggets on the path.
What remains above all
is a sense of marvel and gratitude.

Combustible

Benign spirits modulate my emotions
so that centrifugal fears and furies
sucking at me from within
can be released or transformed.

But if one day
the devil rides my bumper,
aggravating me with white-hot insults
will I spew fumes like an overheated engine
or will I be able to shift into neutral
and coast back into balanced tranquility
with a steady hand of wisdom at the wheel?

You Could Be Wrong

Illness shall have no dominion
over your healthy body.
But you could be wrong.

You believe in the power of your thoughts
to split clouds, make rain.
But you could be wrong.

The Lord is your shepherd,
you are safe in his flock.
But you could be wrong.

You feel that your eyes are unfailing,
spying secrets beneath the surface.
But you could be wrong.

You build your house on a rock,
it cannot crumble.
But you could be wrong.

The wind bloweth
where it listeth,
and the wind could be right.

Living Deferred

Afraid of life
I hid in a dark closet,
plugging my ears with my thumbs
and burying my face between my knees.
I shuddered during sleepless nights
when my heart heard the moans of the hungry.
My skin prickled
when tears of grief rained down on me
through the cracks in the wall.
And I recoiled from my imagination,
alarmed by ghosts from ages past.

Only when I dared to strike out
and travel along ordinary roads
where pebbles bruised my feet
and thorns stuck my fingers,
when I broke bread with a stranger
and held hands with a bereft companion,
and where even the spirits of the deceased
hovered peacefully nearby in their twilight zone
--only then could I tame my worries,
and begin to live.

Ute Carson

A Guest at a Wedding

Just back from greeting her first grandchild,
my friend Elsa said, "In the midst of all the joy
I felt like a guest at a wedding."
Aren't we all guests in our relationships,
maybe special guests, honored guests, but still guests?
Sometimes we become hosts
sitting at the head of the table
with a bride, a groom, a glowing new parent.
But mostly we are guests among other guests,
looking on and sharing life's events.

The Lure of the Ordinary

When we first met
we were surging toward separate shores.
When did we start moving to the music of the water?
Was it while propped
against the headboard of our bed,
books resting in our laps?
Or fingering figures on each others' backs
before falling asleep?
Or wordlessly sharing
the calm after lovemaking?
As all things long established
fall into a rhythm,
we too are lulled
by the ebb and flow of the ordinary.

Sunrise, Sunset

We tumble into life
and during our journey
we often stumble and fall.
First there is dependency
when we need tending and nurture.
Then the path forks,
one life echoes another
and we become equals in a caring community.
With age independence wanes
as we prepare for our departure,
hoping for a cushioned landing
into the arms of those
who first cared for us.

Success

It takes effort to inflate the balloon of success
which occasionally floats beyond one's expectations.
Hold the tether gently between thumb and finger,
then look up at the gorgeous ball and savor it...
like the full moon in all its splendor
only briefly before it wanes.

Mystery

Many things I do not understand.
Life's meaning often eludes me.
But when I watch the sun set over the sea,
slip slowly from golden glow
to honeyed hue,
then morph into a flaming fireball
before dipping suddenly
into deep blue water,
leaving flamingo pink traces on the clouds,
I gaze in awe at this mysterious oracle.

A Tangled Nest of Moments

The Mysteries of Others

Our thoughts drift away with the clouds
but we can pull them back down at will.
We squirrel away our emotions in the unconscious
and dig them up again when needed.
Often the thoughts and feelings of others elude us,
sifting through gaps in our understanding
like flour through the mesh of a sieve.
I huddle in my dead mother's sweater,
her scent still clinging to the fabric
but her presence forever evades me.
The touch of my lover is on my body,
but I wonder about his fantasies.
I am spellbound by my grandmother's tales
of growing up in a castle
and I wish in vain that I could experience her past.
In his dreams my grandson gathers stones and sticks,
and a green frog hops onto his outstretched palm,
but I cannot follow him to his hideouts.
I hear accounts of terrible pain,
hunger, loss and confinement.
I cannot stretch my sympathies
and feel what those sufferers endure.
I am like a spy, my ear pressed against a wall.
I hear whispers and laughter,
I catch the word "Stop." Lovers teasing, quarreling?
I see two old men playing cards.
I gather snippets of facts, storylines,
and try to relate them to my own emotions
but all I end up with are guesses, surmises.
Little will I ever know of the mysteries of others.

Boarding School

Mother and daughter hug,
and hug again,
tears streaming down their faces.
Angela tears herself away,
walks through the door to the waiting car.
She waves until the school building
vanishes like a fata morgana.
She has the urge to turn back.
Who will say the healing words "Heile, heile Segen"
over a scraped knee?
Will someone be there to hold her beloved child
when she is distressed?
At last Angela sinks into the plush upholstery of the car,
comforted that her love will remain with her daughter
and that life will guide her in its unique way,
as it should be.

Ute Carson

A Tangled Nest of Moments

Our memories are in the weave.
Ragged bits of cloth threaded around wispy twigs,
scattered leaves and
tattered down furnish the padding.
A lot of refurbishing is needed
after the ravages of winter,
plugging a hole here,
mending unraveled bedding there.

Love is in the fabric.
When first your breath blew back my hair,
chirping baby lips were my music,
and a daughter's tender finger grazed my cheeks.

Near perfection is in the tending.
As the wind whistles around our little abode
we huddle feather-to-feather,
knotting more memories
into our tangled nest of moments.

Toward Evening

In the late afternoon
the shadows are longest
and they trail behind me like regrets,
mournful and dark,
shackled to my ankles,
pulling me back to my past.

Then morning comes
and I fix my gaze
on the tendrils of the sun
illuminating the ruts
in the long road ahead,
away from bondage
toward possibility and hope.

Ute Carson

Before the Traces Are Lost

Each family needs a historian
who records the individual stories,
complete with beginnings and endings,
then connects these separate lives
like links in a chain,
held together by others.

In My End Is My Beginning

I have traveled the world
and felt at home in many places.
But when I stood on the wide steps
of my grandparents' former home
in pre-war Pomerania
I trembled with recognition and recollection.
The spirit of this old villa had somehow
seeped into my bloodstream.
Memories flooded in,
childhood stories came alive,
my hair was seaweed-silky,
and my skin amber-tanned.
I was born here in 1940
before the Soviet army came through.
Only the cathedral and a few neighborhoods
survived the war.

I will die and be buried in a faraway country
among people I love now.
But perhaps from time to time my soul may wing its way
back to the Pomeranian sand dunes
to frolic among the whitecaps
of the blue Baltic Sea where my journey began.

Ute Carson

Letting Go of the Past

She stands in front of the old house
of a former lover who died years ago.
It has new owners, fresh paint.
But the creaky, worn-down wooden steps
remember jubilant young lovers
bounding up to a room where,
in each other's arms on soft bedding
they spun dreams of their future.
She brings the memory to mind,
holds it there briefly, savors it,
and then, smiling, walks on.

Carpe Diem

"I am alive," the old woman intones.
Her past is like a valued instrument
she learned to play through joy and tribulation.
She aims to create new melodies in the future.
But for now she sings "seize the day,"
not knowing how long the music will last.

Give Me One More Time

The air is cherry-blossom scented,
such a pleasant ride.
I want to turn the next corner,
and the next, and still one more,
to the mirth of a wedding,
delight in a great-grandchild,
my hand stroking a horse's coat,
and to a fall meadow
where my lover and I had lain
like two rust-colored matted leaves.

Thus fully nourished,
will I beg for more time,
or will I ask to be let off
at the next stop, knowing
that it is my final destination.

The Waters Within

The rhythm of my life emerged from the Baltic Sea
where waves washed over my squealing body
and my toddler feet slogged through sand
studded with honeyed amber
and my plump baby arms
reached out to seagulls,
their wings dipping in and out
of the blue-green water.

Today I swim like a frog,
head above the surface, paddling,
my eyes scanning the sea, flashing like silver.
But the rhythm of the ocean lives within me
as cycles of sun and moon live within me.
Within, I glide on swells to the far horizon,
out of sight, and then float back
with the sea-foam breaking onto the shore.

The ocean rises and falls,
pregnant with new possibilities,
and I am lulled
by the eternal recurrence of the tides.

Ute Carson

About the Author

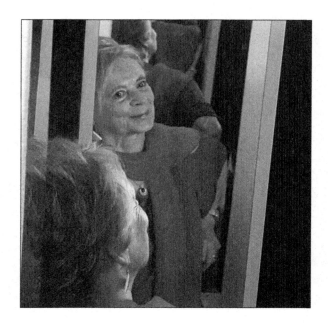

A writer from youth and an M.A. graduate in comparative literature from the University of Rochester, German-born Ute Carson published her first prose piece in 1977. *Colt Tailing*, a 2004 novel, was a finalist for the Peter Taylor Book Award. Carson's story "The Fall" won Outrider Press's Grand Prize and appeared in its short story and poetry anthology *A Walk through My Garden*, 2007. Her second novel, *In Transit*, was published in 2008. Her poems have appeared in numerous journals and magazines in the US and abroad. Carson's poetry was featured on the televised *Spoken Word Showcase* 2009, 2010 and 2011, Channel Austin, Texas. A poetry collection, *Just a Few Feathers* was published in 2011. The poem "A Tangled Nest of Moments" placed second in the Eleventh International Poetry Competition 2012. Her chapbook *Folding Washing* was published in 2013 and her collection of poems *My Gift to Life* was nominated for the 2015 Pushcart Award Prize. *Save the Last Kiss*, a novella, was published in 2016.

Ute Carson resides in Austin, Texas with her husband. They have three daughters, six grandchildren, a horse and a clowder of cats.

Visit her website at www.utecarson.com

CPSIA information can be obtained
at www.ICGtesting.com
Printed in the USA
LVOW13s1530200318

570510LV00003B/69/P

9 781632 100320